# THE DEFINITIVE PLANT BASED DIET COOKBOOK

A Complete cookbook with tasty and wholesome recipes to lose weight in a few steps. Lose weight fast while eating tasty foods.

**Ursa Males**

# TABLE OF CONTENTS

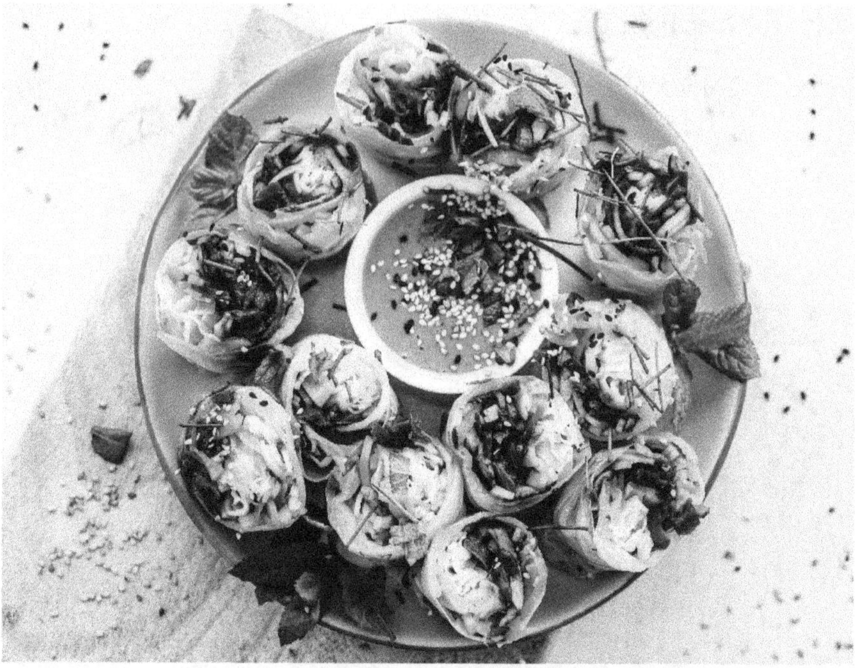

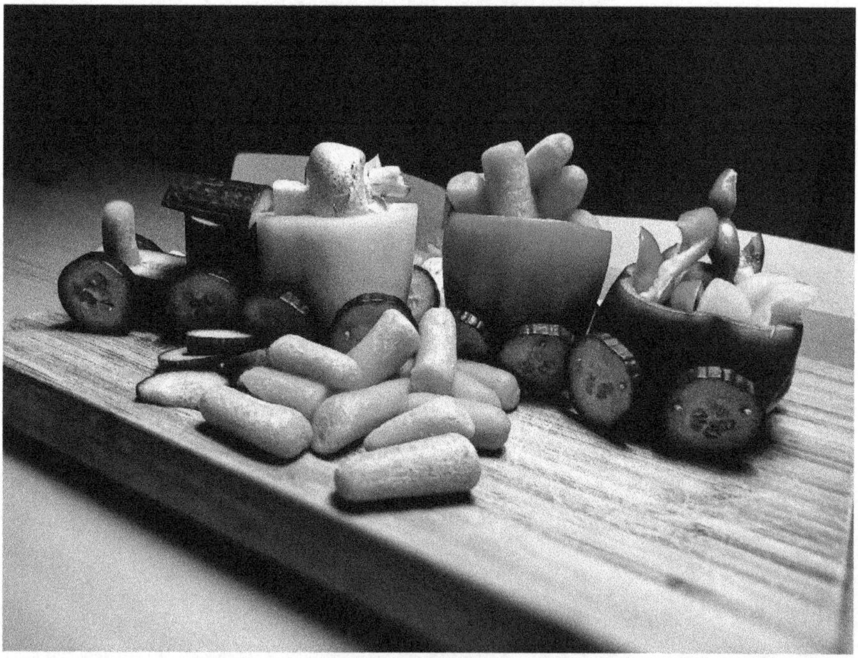

# BREAKFAST

## 1. The Fruit Smoothie Formula

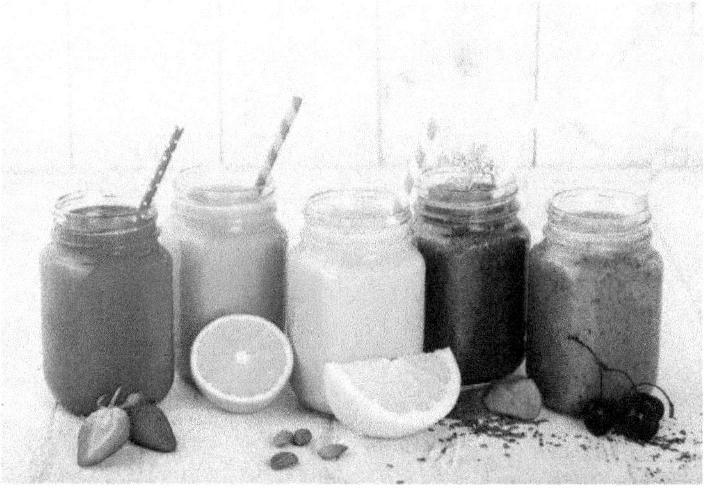

Preparation time: 5 minutes

Cooking time: 0 minutes

Servings: 2

**Ingredients**:

- 2 cups unsweetened plant milk
- 2 cups chopped fresh or frozen fruit
- 2 tablespoons ground flaxseed
- 1 cup ice (optional, if using fresh fruit)

**Directions:**

1. Combine all the fixings in a blender and purée for 30 seconds to 1 minute, until smooth and creamy.

**Nutrition:** Calories: 253 Fat: 8g Protein: 10gCarbs: 39g

## 2. Avocado and 'Sausage' Breakfast Sandwich

Preparation Time: 15 minutes

Cooking Time: 10 minutes

Servings: 1

**Ingredients:**

- 1 vegan sausage patty
- 1 cup kale, chopped
- 2 teaspoons extra virgin olive oil
- 1 tablespoon pepitas
- Salt and pepper, to taste
- 1 tablespoon vegan mayo
- 1/8 teaspoon chipotle powder
- 1 teaspoon jalapeno chopped
- 1 English muffin, toasted
- ¼ avocado, sliced

**Directions**:

1. Place a sauté pan over high heat and add a drop of oil. Add the vegan patty and cook for 2 minutes. Flip the patty, then add the kale and pepitas.
2. Season well, then cook for another few minutes until the patty is cooked. Find a small bowl and add the mayo, chipotle powder, and jalapeno. Stir well to combine.
3. Place the muffin onto a flat surface, spread with the spicy mayo, then top with the patty.

4. Add the sliced avocado, then serve and enjoy.

**Nutrition:** Calories: 573 Fat: 23g Carbs: 36g Protein: 21g

## 3. <u>Cinnamon Rolls with Cashew Frosting</u>

Preparation Time: 25 minutes

Cooking Time: 25 minutes

Servings: 12

**Ingredients:**

- 3 tablespoons vegan butter
- ¾ cup unsweetened almond milk
- ½ teaspoon salt
- 3 tablespoons caster sugar
- 1 teaspoon vanilla extract
- ½ cup pumpkin puree
- 3 cups all-purpose flour
- 2 ¼ teaspoons dried active yeast
- 3 tablespoons softened vegan butter
- 3 tablespoons brown sugar
- ½ teaspoon cinnamon
- ½ cup cashews
- ½ cup icing sugar
- 1 teaspoon vanilla extract
- 2/3 cup almond milk

**Directions:**

1. Soak the cashews for 1 hour in boiling water. Grease a baking sheet and pop to one side. Find a small bowl, add the butter, and pop into the microwave to melt.

2. Add the sugar and stir well, then set aside to cool. Grab a large bowl and add the flour, salt, and yeast. Stir well to mix.
3. Place the cooled butter into a jug, add the pumpkin puree, vanilla, and almond milk. Stir well together. Pour the wet fixings into the dry and stir well to combine.
4. Tip onto a flat surface and knead for 5 minutes, adding extra flour as needed to avoid sticking. Pop back into the bowl, cover with plastic wrap and pop into the fridge overnight.
5. Remove the dough from the fridge and punch down with your fingers. Using a rolling pin, roll to form an 18" rectangle, then spread with butter.
6. Find a small bowl and add the sugar and cinnamon. Mix well, then sprinkle with the butter. Roll the dough into a large sausage, then slice into sections.
7. Place onto the greased baking sheet and leave in a dark place to rise for one hour—Preheat the oven to 350°F. Strain the cashews and put them in your blender. Whizz until smooth.
8. Add the sugar and the vanilla, then whizz again. Add the almond milk until it reaches your desired consistency.
9. Pop into the oven and bake for 20 minutes until golden. Pour the glaze over the top, then serve and enjoy.

**Nutrition:** Calories: 243 Fat: 9g Carbs: 34g Protein: 4g

## 4. <u>Vegan Variety Poppy Seed Scones</u>

Preparation Time: 5 minutes

Cooking Time: 10 minutes

Servings: 12.

**Ingredients:**

- 1 cup white sugar
- 2 cups flour
- Juice from 1 lemon
- Zest from 1 lemon
- 4 teaspoon baking powder
- ½ teaspoon salt
- 1 cup Earth Balance or vegan butter
- 2 tablespoon poppy seeds
- ½ cup soymilk
- 1/3 cup water

**Directions:**

1. Warm oven to 400°F. Next, mix the sugar, the flour, the powder, and the salt in a big mixing bowl.
2. Add the vegan butter to the mixture and cut it up until you create a sand-like mixture. Next, add the lemon juice, the lemon zest, and the poppy seeds. Add the water and the soy milk, and stir the ingredients well.
3. Portion the batter out over a baking sheet in about ¼ cup portions.

4. Allow the scones to bake for fifteen minutes and let them cool before serving. Enjoy.

**Nutrition:** Calories: 205 Fat: 3g Carbs: 12g Protein: 6g

## 5. Sweet Pomegranate Porridge

Preparation Time: 5 minutes

Cooking Time: 20 minutes

Servings: 4

**Ingredients:**

- 2 cups oats
- 1 ½ cups water
- 1 ½ cups pomegranate juice
- 2 tablespoons Pomegranate Molasses

**Directions:**

1. Pour all fixings into the instant pot and mix well. Seal the lid, and cook on high pressure for four minutes. Use a quick release, and serve warm.

**Nutrition:** Calories: 177 Fat: 6g Carbs: 23g Protein: 8g

## 6. Apple Oatmeal

Preparation Time: 5 minutes

Cooking Time: 20 minutes

Servings: 4

**Ingredients:**

- ¼ teaspoon of sea salt
- 1 cup cashew milk
- 1 cup strawberries, halved & fresh
- 1 tablespoon brown sugar
- 2 cups apples, diced
- 3 cups of water
- ¼ teaspoon coconut oil
- ½ cup steel cut oats

**Directions:**

1. Start by greasing your instant pot with oil, and add everything to it except for the milk and berries.
2. Cook on high pressure within ten minutes. Then add in your milk and strawberries after a natural pressure release. Mix well, and serve warm.

**Nutrition:** Calories: 435 Fat: 7g Carbs: 34g Protein: 8g

## 7. Breakfast Cookies

Preparation Time: 10 minutes

Cooking Time: 6 minutes

Servings: 24-32

**Ingredients:**

Dry Ingredients:

- ½ teaspoon baking powder
- 2 cups rolled oats
- ½ teaspoon baking soda

Wet Ingredients:

- 1 teaspoon pure vanilla extract
- 2 flax eggs (2 tbsp ground flaxseed & around 6 tablespoons of water, mix and put aside for 15 minutes)
- 2 tablespoons melted coconut oil
- 2 tablespoons pure maple syrup
- ½ cup natural creamy peanut butter
- 2 ripe bananas

Add-in Ingredients:

- ½ cup finely chopped walnuts
- ½ cup raisins

Optional Topping:

- 2 tablespoons chopped walnuts
- 2 tablespoons raisins

**Directions:**

1. Warm oven to 325°F, use parchment paper to line a baking sheet, and put it aside.
2. Put the bananas to a large bowl, and then use a fork to mash them until smooth. Add in the other wet ingredients and mix until well incorporated.
3. Add the dry ingredients and then use a rubber spatula to stir and fold them into the dry ingredients until well mixed. Stir in the walnuts and raisins.
4. Spoon the cookie dough onto your prepared baking sheet, ensuring that you leave adequate space between the cookies.
5. Bake in the preheated oven for around 12 minutes. Once ready, let the cookies cool on the baking sheet for around 10 minutes.
6. Lift the cookies carefully from the baking sheet onto a cooling rack to further cool.

**Nutrition:** Calories: 565 Fat: 6g Carbs: 32g Protein: 8g

# LUNCH

## 8. Barbecued Greens & Grits

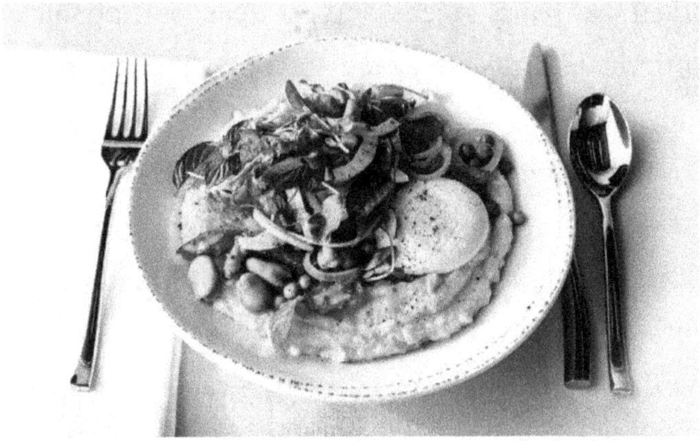

Preparation time: 60 minutes

Cooking time: 35 minutes

Servings: 4

**Ingredients:**

- 1 14-oz. package tempeh, cut into slices
- 3 cups vegetable broth
- 3 cups collard greens, chopped
- ½ cup BBQ sauce
- 1 cup gluten-free grits
- ¼ cup white onion, diced
- 2 tbsp. olive oil
- 2 garlic cloves, minced
- 1 tsp. salt

**Directions:**

1. Preheat the oven to 400°F. Mix tempeh it with the BBQ sauce in a shallow baking dish. Set aside and let marinate for up to 3 hours. Heat 1 tbsp. Put olive oil in a frying pan, then add the garlic and sauté until fragrant.
2. Add the collard greens and ½ Teaspoon of salt and cook until the collards are wilted and dark. Remove from the heat and set aside.
3. Cover the tempeh and BBQ sauce mixture with aluminum foil—Bake in the oven the ingredients for 15 minutes. Uncover and continue to bake within another 10 minutes until the tempeh is browned and crispy.
4. While the tempeh cooks, heat the remaining tablespoon of olive oil in the previously used frying pan over medium heat. Cook the onions until brown and fragrant, around 10 minutes.
5. Put in the vegetable broth and boil; then turn the heat down to low. Slowly whisk the grits into the simmering broth. Add the remaining ½ Teaspoon of salt before covering the pan with a lid.
6. Let the ingredients simmer for about 8 minutes until the grits are soft and creamy. Serve the tempeh and collard greens on top of a bowl of grits and enjoy, or store for later!

**Nutrition:** Calories: 394Carbs: 39.3 g Fat: 17.6 g Protein: 19.7 g.

## 9. Greens and Olives Pan

Preparation time: 10 minutes

Cooking time: 15 minutes

Servings: 4

**Ingredients:**

- 4 spring onions, chopped
- 2 tablespoons olive oil
- ½ cup green olives pitted and halved
- ¼ cup pine nuts, toasted
- 1 tablespoon balsamic vinegar
- 2 cups baby spinach
- 1 cup baby arugula
- 1 cup asparagus, trimmed, blanched, and halved
- Salt and black pepper to the taste

**Directions:**

1. Heat-up a pan with the oil over medium-high heat, add the spring onions and the asparagus, and sauté for 5 minutes.
2. Add the olives, spinach, and the other ingredients, toss, cook over medium heat for 10 minutes, divide between plates and serve for lunch.

**Nutrition:** Calories 136Fat 13.1gCarbs 4.4gProtein 2.8g

## 10. Mushrooms and Chard Soup

Preparation time: 10 minutes

Cooking time: 30 minutes

Servings: 4

**Ingredients:**

- 3 cups Swiss chard, chopped
- 6 cups vegetable stock
- 1 cup mushrooms, sliced
- 2 garlic cloves, minced
- 1 tablespoon olive oil
- 2 scallions, chopped
- 2 tablespoons balsamic vinegar
- ¼ cup basil, chopped
- Salt and black pepper to the taste
- 1 tablespoon cilantro, chopped

**Directions:**

1. Heat-up a pot with the oil over medium-high heat, add the scallions and the garlic, and sauté for 5 minutes. Add the mushrooms and sauté for another 5 minutes.
2. Add the rest of the ingredients, toss, bring to a simmer and cook over medium heat for 20 minutes more.

3. Ladle the soup into bowls and serve.

**Nutrition:** Calories 140Fat 4gCarbs 4gProtein 8g

## 11. Tomato, Green Beans, and Chard Soup

Preparation time: 10 minutes

Cooking time: 35 minutes

Servings: 4

**Ingredients:**

- 2 scallions, chopped
- 1 cup swiss chard, chopped
- 1 tablespoon olive oil
- 1 red bell pepper, chopped
- salt and black pepper to the taste
- 1 cup tomatoes, cubed
- 1 cup green beans, chopped
- 6 cups vegetable stock
- 2 tablespoons tomato passata
- 2 garlic cloves, minced
- 2 teaspoons thyme, chopped
- ½ teaspoon red pepper flakes

**Directions:**

1. Heat-up a pot with the oil over medium heat, add the scallions, garlic, pepper flakes, and sauté for 5 minutes.
2. Add the chard and the other ingredients, toss, bring to a simmer and cook over medium heat for 30 minutes more.

3. Ladle the soup into bowls and serve for lunch.

**Nutrition:** Calories 150Fat 8gCarbs 4gProtein 9g

## 12. Hot Roasted Peppers Cream

Preparation time: 10 minutes

Cooking time: 30 minutes

Servings: 4

**Ingredients:**

- 1 red chili pepper, minced
- 4 garlic cloves, minced
- 2 pounds mixed bell peppers, roasted, peeled, and chopped
- 4 scallions, chopped
- 1 cup coconut cream
- Salt and black pepper to the taste
- 2 tablespoons olive oil
- ½ tablespoon basil, chopped
- 4 cups vegetable stock
- ¼ cup chives, chopped

**Directions:**

1. Warm-up a pot with the oil on medium heat, put the garlic and the chili pepper, and sauté for 5 minutes.
2. Add the peppers and the other ingredients, toss, bring to a simmer and cook over medium heat for 25 minutes.

3. Blend the soup using an immersion blender, divide into bowls and serve.

**Nutrition:** Calories 140 Fat 2g Carbs 5g Protein 8g

## 13. Eggplant and Peppers Soup

Preparation time: 10 minutes

Cooking time: 40 minutes

Servings: 4

**Ingredients:**

- 2 red bell peppers, chopped
- 3 scallions, chopped
- 3 garlic cloves, minced
- 2 tablespoon olive oil
- Salt and black pepper to the taste
- 5 cups vegetable stock
- 1 bay leaf
- ½ cup coconut cream
- 1-pound eggplants, roughly cubed
- 2 tablespoons basil, chopped

**Directions:**

1. Warm-up your pot with the oil on medium heat, put the scallions and the garlic, and sauté for 5 minutes. Add the peppers and the eggplants and sauté for 5 minutes more.
2. Add the remaining ingredients, toss, bring to a simmer, cook for 30 minutes, ladle into bowls and serve for lunch.

**Nutrition:** Calories 180Fat 2gCarbs 5gProtein 10g

## 14. Eggplant and Olives Stew

Preparation time: 10 minutes

Cooking time: 30 minutes

Servings: 4

**Ingredients:**

- 2 scallions, chopped
- 2 tablespoons avocado oil
- 2 garlic cloves, chopped
- 1 bunch parsley, chopped
- Salt and black pepper to the taste
- 1 teaspoon basil, dried
- 1 teaspoon cumin, dried
- 2 eggplants, roughly cubed
- 1 cup green olives, pitted and sliced
- 3 tablespoons balsamic vinegar
- ½ Cup tomato passata

**Directions:**

1. Warm-up your pot with the oil on medium heat, put the scallions, garlic, basil, cumin, and sauté for 5 minutes.
2. Add the eggplants and the other ingredients, toss, cook over medium heat for 25 minutes more, divide into bowls and serve.

**Nutrition:** Calories 93Fat 1.8gCarbs 18.6gProtein 3.4g

# DINNER

## 15. Stuffed Zucchini

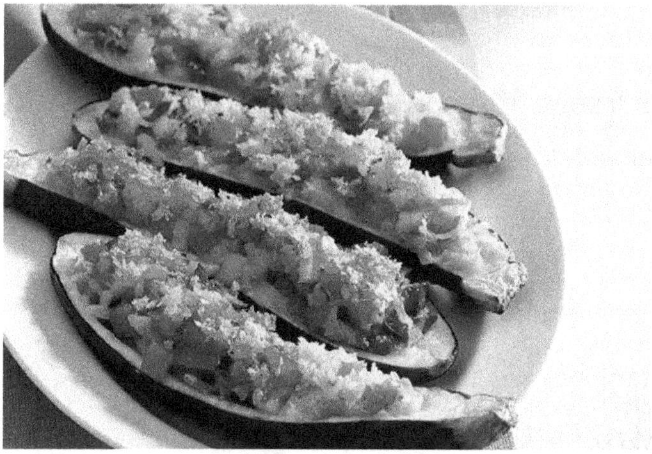

Preparation time: 15 minutes

Cooking time: 25 minutes

Servings: 4

**Ingredients:**

- 1 ½ cup black beans, drained
- ¼ tsp chili powder

½ of the following:

- sea salt
- cumin, ground
- 1 tsp of the following:
- clove garlic, minced

- red bell pepper, diced
- red onion, diced
- 1 tbsp. olive oil, extra virgin
- 4 medium zucchinis

For the Sauce:

¼ tsp of the following:

- chili powder
- turmeric
- sea salt
- 1 tbsp. Nutritional yeast
- ½ tsp apple cider vinegar

¼ cup of the following:

- water
- raw tahini
- 4 tsp Lemon juice

**Directions:**

1. Set the oven to 350 heat setting. Slice the knobs off the top and bottom of the zucchini, and then slice in half lengthwise.
2. Scoop the center of the seeds from each zucchini with a spoon, creating a bowl to hold the filling. On a big cookie sheet, place the zucchini bowls and bake for approximately 20 minutes.
3. Using a big skillet, combine onion and pepper and sauté for five minutes at medium-high temperature until softened. Add garlic and sauté for an additional minute.

4. Turn the skillet down to medium heat and sprinkle in the chili powder, cumin, salt, and black beans and warm. Remove from the stove and cover to maintain warmth.
5. Prepare the sauce. Using a little bowl, whisk the sauce ingredients until smooth and creamy. Remove the zucchini from the oven when finished cooking.
6. Fill each zucchini bowl generously with the bean mixture. Drizzle the sauce over. Serve warm and enjoy!

**Nutrition**: Calories: 159 Carbohydrates: 8 g Proteins: 26 g Fats: 2 g

## 16. Roasted Butternut Squash with Chimichurri

Preparation time: 15 minutes

Cooking time: 15 minutes

Servings: 2

**Ingredients:**

- 1 cup onion, thinly sliced
- 2 cloves garlic
- 1 tbsp. coconut oil
- 1 acorn squash
- 2 tbsp. olive oil (best if extra virgin)
- ¼ cup goji berries
- 1 cup water
- 2 cups mushrooms, sliced
- ½ cup quinoa

Chimichurri Sauce:

- ½ tsp salt
- 2 tbsp. lime
- ½ cup olive oil, extra virgin
- ¼ tsp cayenne pepper
- 1 shallot
- 3 cloves garlic
- 1 tbsp. sherry vinegar
- 1 cup parsley

**Directions:**

1. Bring the broiler to the maximum heat setting. Stir up the chimichurri sauce by combining the parsley, vinegar, garlic shallot, cayenne pepper, olive oil, lime juice, and ½ cup of olive oil.
2. Blend well; if you want the sauce a little thinner, then add additional extra virgin oil. Prepare an aluminum-foiled cookie sheet.
3. Divide the squash in half by carefully cutting widthwise, and remove seeds and pulp from the center. Cut each half of the squash into moon shape slices; you should get about 4-6 slices.
4. Place the slices on the aluminum foil sheet and spritz olive oil across the top. Once one side is charred to your liking, flip the squash and char the other side.
5. While broiling, bring a medium-sized saucepan of water to a rolling boil then simmer the quinoa, cooking for 10 minutes or until tender.
6. Heat a skillet to medium heat, and sauté the onions. Once the onions are caramelizing, add in the mushroom and garlic, cooking on low heat for approximately 5 minutes.
7. Plate the squash, topping it with quinoa and mushroom. Sprinkle goji berries across the plate and drizzle chimichurri sauce.

8. Serve warm and enjoy!

**Nutrition:** Calories: 615 Carbohydrates: 71.6 g Proteins: 12.5 g Fats: 35.7 g

## 17. <u>Eggplant Pizza</u>

Preparation time: 15 minutes

Cooking time: 30 minutes

Servings: 8

**Ingredients:**

- 2 tbsp. olive oil

¼ tsp of the following:

- pepper
- salt
- ½ tsp oregano, dried
- 1 cup panko
- ½ tbsp. almond flour
- 1 tbsp. flaxseed, ground
- 1/3 cup water
- ½ eggplant, medium size
- 2 cups marinara sauce
- 1 lb. vegan pizza dough

For the cheese:

- ¼ lb. tofu, extra firm drained
- 2 tbsp. almond milk, unsweetened
- ½ cup cashews, soaked for 6 hours, drained
- 3 tbsp. lemon juice, freshly squeezed

**Directions:**

1. Set the oven to 400 heat setting; prepare a cookie sheet with ½ tablespoon of olive oil by brushing to coat. Whisk together flaxseed, flour, and water in a little bowl.
2. In a different bowl, combine salt, pepper, oregano, and panko. Prepare the eggplant by slicing into ¼ inch triangles.
3. Dip each eggplant triangle into the flaxseed mixture then coat with panko mixture and place on the cookie sheet.
4. Slide gently into the oven and baking for 15 minutes. Flip and then bake for an additional 15 minutes or until lightly browned.
5. Take out of the oven and set to the side. Get a pizza stone or pizza pan ready for the dough.
6. Lightly flour the workspace, and with a rolling pin, work the dough to a 14-inch circle then transfer to the pizza stone or pizza pan.
7. Brush the dough's top with olive oil and slide into the warm oven, cooking until lightly browned or for about twenty minutes.
8. While the crust is baking, prepare the cheese by placing cashews in the high-speed blender, blending until it reaches a crumbly consistency.
9. Then add to the blender the lemon juice, almond milk, and tofu; blend until it's a chunky cheese-like consistency. Set to the side.
10. Once the crust is cooked, assemble the pizza by saucing crust with marinara, adding eggplant slices, and placing the cheese on top.

11. Serve warm and enjoy!

**Nutrition:** Calories: 234 Carbohydrates: 27 g Proteins: 5.4 g Fats: 12 g

## 18. Green Avocado Carbonara

Preparation time: 15 minutes

Cooking time: 0 minutes

Servings: 1

**Ingredients:**

- Spinach angel hair
- Parsley, fresh
- 2 tsp olive oil, extra virgin
- 2 cloves garlic, diced
- ½ lemon, zest, and juice
- 1 avocado, pitted
- Salt and pepper to taste

**Directions**:

1. Combine using a food processor the parsley, olive oil, garlic, lemon, and avocado and blend until smooth. Prepare the noodles according to package.
2. Place noodles in a bowl, and add the sauce on top of noodles. Add pepper and salt to your liking. Serve warm and enjoy!

**Nutrition:** Calories: 526 Carbohydrates: 24.6 g Proteins: 5.8 g Fats: 48.7 g

## 19. Curried Tofu

Preparation time: 15 minutes

Cooking time: 30 minutes

Servings: 4

**Ingredients:**

- ¼ tsp garlic powder
- 2 tbsp. curry powder
- 1 pack extra firm tofu

**Directions:**

1. Heat to 400 degrees the oven. Slice the tofu into cubes. Put the garlic powder, curry powder, and cubed tofu in a container with a lid.
2. Close it tightly and shake lightly just to coat the tofu. Make sure there's even coverage of the spices.
3. On a parchment-lined cookie sheet, place the tofu cubes and bake for 15 minutes, flip and continue baking for another 15 minutes or until crisp. Serve warm and enjoy!

**Nutrition:** Calories: 345 Carbohydrates: 37 g Proteins: 33.9 g Fats: 6.3 g

## 20. Sesame Tofu and Eggplant

Preparation time: 15 minutes

Cooking time: 10 minutes

Servings: 4

**Ingredients:**

- 1 tbsp. olive oil
- ¼ cup of the following:
- sesame seeds
- soy sauce
- 1 eggplant
- 1 pound firm tofu
- 1 tsp crushed red pepper flakes
- 2 cloves garlic
- 2 tsp sweetener of your choice
- 4 tbsp. toasted sesame oil
- 1 cup cilantro, chopped
- 3 tbsp. rice vinegar
- Salt and pepper to taste

**Directions**:

1. Set the oven to 200 heat setting. Blot the tofu using paper towels to absorb excess moisture.
2. In a big mixing bowl, whisk together red pepper flakes, garlic, sesame oil, vinegar, and ¼ cup of cilantro to create the marinade.

3. With a mandolin, julienne the eggplant. If you do not have this, you can create the noodles by hand. Mix the noodles in the big bowl with the marinade.
4. Add oil to a skillet over medium-low flame setting, and cook the eggplant until soft.
5. Turn off the oven, and add the last of the cilantro.
6. Transfer the contents from the skillet to an oven-safe dish, cover with foil, and place in the oven to keep warm. Cut the tofu into 8 slices and coat with sesame seeds. Press the sesame seeds into the tofu.
7. In the skillet, add 2 tablespoons of sesame oil and warm under medium heat. Fry the tofu for 5 minutes then flip and fry.
8. Pour the soy sauce into the pan, coating the tofu. Cook until the tofu looks caramelized.
9. Remove the noodles and plate with the tofu on top of the noodles. Serve warm and enjoy!

**Nutrition:** Calories: 295 Carbohydrates: 6.87 g Proteins: 11.21 g Fats: 6.87 g

## 21. Tempeh Coconut Curry

Preparation time: 15 minutes

Cooking time: 25 minutes

Servings: 4

**Ingredients**:

Curry:

2 tsp of the following:

- low-sodium soy sauce
- tamarind pulp

1 tbsp. of the following:

- lime juice
- garlic, finely chopped
- ginger, finely chopped
- vegetable oil
- salt
- 8 oz. tempeh
- 13 1/2 oz. coconut milk, light
- 1 cup water
- 3 cups sweet potato, chopped
- 1 cinnamon stick

½ tsp of the following:

- red pepper, crushed
- turmeric, ground
- 1 ½ tsp coriander, ground

- 2 cups onion, finely chopped

Rice:

- 1 ½ cup cauliflower rice
- ¼ tsp salt
- 1/3 cup cilantro, chopped

**Directions:**

1. Using a medium-high heat setting, warm some oil in a big pot or whatever you prefer, as long as it's nonstick. Place the onion and ½ teaspoon of salt and sauté for approximately 2 minutes.
2. Next, stir in the tamarind, breaking it up as you combine in the skillet and cooking for another 2 minutes.
3. Add in the ginger, garlic, coriander, turmeric, crushed red pepper, and cinnamon stick; stir constantly.
4. Add in the additional salt, tempeh, milk, water, and potatoes, bringing to a boil. Cover, allowing to simmer within 15 minutes or until tender.
5. Mix in the soy sauce then simmer for 3 additional minutes. Remove the cinnamon stick. Cook the cauliflower rice according to package instructions.
6. Stir in the cilantro. Place the rice in a bowl and cover with curry. Serve warm and enjoy!

**Nutrition:** Calories: 558 Carbohydrates: 54.2 g Proteins: 18.4 g Fats: 33.5 g

# SNACKS

## 22. Beans with Sesame Hummus

Preparation time: 10 minutes

Cooking time: 0 minutes

Servings: 6

**Ingredients:**

- 4 tbsp sesame oil
- 2 cloves garlic finely sliced
- 1 can (15 oz) cannellini beans, drained
- 4 tbsp sesame paste
- 2 tbsp lemon juice freshly squeezed
- 1/4 tsp red pepper flakes
- 2 tbsp fresh basil finely chopped
- 2 tbsp fresh parsley finely chopped
- sea salt to taste

**Directions:**

1. Place all ingredients in your food processor. Process until all ingredients are combined well and smooth. Transfer mixture into a bowl and refrigerate until servings.

**Nutrition:** Calories: 80 Carbs: 5g Fat: 6g Protein: 2g

## 23. Candied Honey-Coconut Peanuts

Preparation time: 15 minutes

Cooking time: 10 minutes

Servings: 8

**Ingredients**

- 1/2 cup honey (preferably a darker honey)
- 4 tbsp coconut butter softened
- 1 tsp ground cinnamon
- 4 cups roasted, salted peanuts

**Directions**

1. Add honey, coconut butter, and cinnamon in a microwave-safe bowl. Microwave at high for about 4 to 5 minutes. Stir in nuts; mix thoroughly to coat.
2. Microwave at high 5 to 6 minutes or until foamy; stir after 3 minutes. Spread in a single layer on a greased tray. Refrigerated for 6 hours. Break into small pieces and serve.

**Nutrition:** Calories: 150 Carbs: 17g Fat: 8g Protein: 3g

## 24. Choco Walnuts Fat Bombs

Preparation time: 15 minutes

Cooking time: 0 minutes

Servings: 6

**Ingredients**

- 1/2 cup coconut butter
- 1/2 cup coconut oil softened
- 4 tbs cocoa powder, unsweetened
- 4 tbs brown sugar firmly packed
- 1/3 cup silken tofu mashed
- 1 cup walnuts, roughly chopped

**Directions**

1. Add coconut butter and coconut oil into a microwave dish; melt it for 10-15 seconds. Add in cocoa powder and whisk well.
2. Pour mixture into a blender with brown sugar and silken tofu cream; blend for 3-4 minutes. Place silicone molds onto a sheet pan and fill halfway with chopped walnuts.
3. Pour the mixture over the walnuts and place it in the freezer for 6 hours. Ready! Serve!

**Nutrition:** Calories: 196 Carbs: 6g Fat: 28g Protein: 3g

## 25. Crispy Honey Pecans

Preparation time: 2 hours and 15 minutes

Cooking time: 3 hours

Servings: 4

**Ingredients:**

- 16 oz pecan halves
- 4 tbsp coconut butter melted
- 4 to 5 tbsp honey strained
- 1/4 tsp ground ginger
- 1/4 tsp ground allspice
- 1 1/2 tsp ground cinnamon

**Directions:**

1. Add pecans and melted coconut butter into your 4-quart Slow Cooker. Stir until combined well. Add in honey and stir well.
2. In a bowl, combine spices and sprinkle over nuts; stir lightly. Cook on low uncovered for about 2 to 3 hours or until nuts are crispy. Serve cold.

**Nutrition:** Calories: 220 Carbs: 29g Fat: 14g Protein: 2g

## 26. Crunchy Fried Pickles

Preparation time: 10 minutes

Cooking time: 5 minutes

Servings: 6

**Ingredients:**

- 1/2 cup Vegetable oil for frying
- 1 cup all-purpose flour
- 1 cup plain breadcrumbs
- Pinch of salt and pepper
- 30 pickle chips (cucumber, dill)

**Directions:**

1. Heat oil in a large frying skillet over medium-high heat. Stir the flour, breadcrumbs, and the salt and pepper in a shallow bowl.
2. Dredge the pickles in the flour/breadcrumbs mixture to coat completely. Fry in batches until golden brown on all sides, 2 to 3 minutes in total. Drain on paper towels and serve.

**Nutrition**: Calories: 287 Carbs: 28g Fat: 19g Protein: 4g

## 27. Turnip Fries

Preparation Time: 25 minutes

Cooking Time: 20 minutes

Servings: 8

**Ingredients:**

- 1 tsp. onion powder
- 1 tsp. paprika
- 1 tsp. garlic salt
- 1 tbsp. vegetable oil
- 3 pounds turnips

**Directions:**

1. Set the oven to 425 heat setting. Prepare a lightly greased aluminum foil-lined cookie sheet
2. Using a hand peeler, peel the turnips. With a Mandolin, cut the turnips into French fry sticks. Then place in a big bowl.
3. Toss the turnips with oil to coat then season with onion powder, paprika, and garlic and coat again. Spread evenly across the cookie sheet.
4. Bake for at least 20 minutes or until the outside is crisp. Serve with your favorite sauce or enjoy alone.

**Nutrition:** Calories: 87 Protein: 5.98 g Fat: 3.15 g Carbohydrates: 8.76 g

## 28. Lime and Chili Carrots Noodles

Preparation Time: 10 minutes

Cooking Time: 0 minutes

Servings: 4

**Ingredients:**

½ tsp of the following:

- Black pepper
- Salt
- 2 tbsp. coconut oil
- ¼ cup coriander, finely chopped
- 2 Jalapeno chilis
- 1 tbsp. lime juice
- 2 carrots, peeled and spiralized

**Directions:**

1. In a little bowl, combine jalapeno, lime juice, and coconut oil to form a sauce. In a big bowl, place the carrot noodles and pour dressing over the top.
2. Toss to ensure the dressing fully coats the noodles. Season with pepper and salt. Serve and enjoy.

**Nutrition:** Calories: 93 Protein: 1.92 g Fat: 8.4 g Carbohydrates: 3.28 g

# VEGETABLES

## 29. Grilled Avocado with Tomatoes

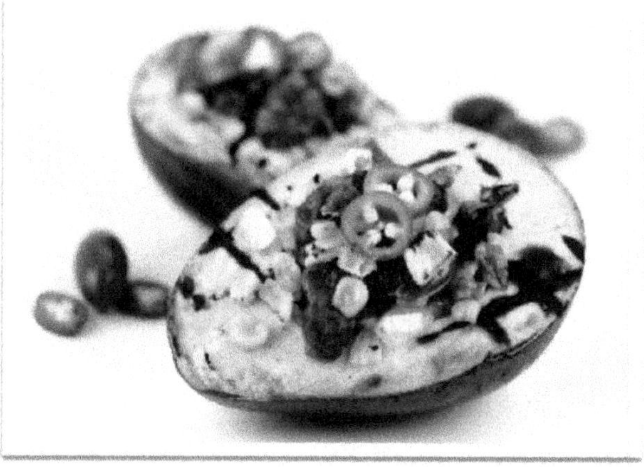

Preparation Time: 10 minutes

Cooking Time: 15 minutes

Servings: 6

**Ingredients:**

- 3 avocados, halved and pitted
- 3 limes, wedged
- 1½ cup grape tomatoes
- 1 cup fresh corn
- 1 cup onion, chopped
- 3 serrano peppers
- 2 garlic cloves, peeled
- ¼ cup cilantro leaves, chopped

- 1 tablespoon olive oil
- Salt and black pepper to taste

**Directions:**

1. Prepare and set a grill over medium heat.
2. Brush the avocado with oil and grill it for 5 minutes per side.
3. Meanwhile, toss the garlic, onion, corn, tomatoes, and pepper in a baking sheet.
4. At 550 degrees F, roast the vegetables for 5 minutes.
5. Toss the veggie mix and stir in salt, cilantro, and black pepper.
6. Mix well then fill the grilled avocadoes with the mixture.
7. Garnish with lime.
8. Serve.

**Nutrition:** Calories: 56Total Fat: 6gCarbs: 3gNet Carbs: 1gFiber: 0g

Protein: 1g

# 30. Grilled Tofu with Chimichurri Sauce

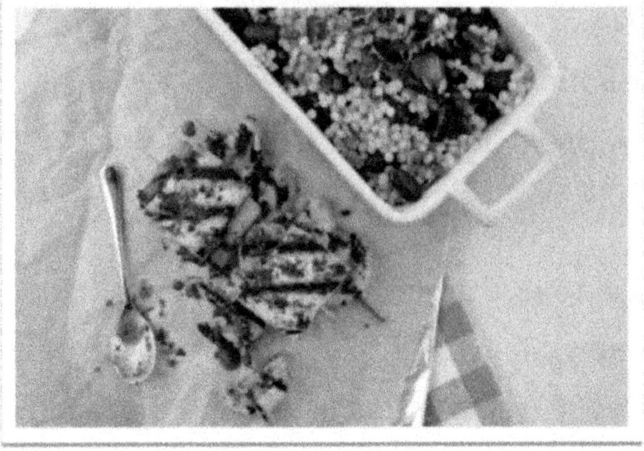

Preparation Time: 10 minutes

Cooking Time: 12 minutes

Servings: 4

**Ingredients**:

- 2 tablespoons plus 1 teaspoon olive oil
- 1 teaspoon dried oregano
- 1 cup parsley leaves
- ½ cup cilantro leaves
- 2 Fresno peppers, seeded and chopped
- 2 tablespoons white wine vinegar
- 2 tablespoons water
- 1 tablespoon fresh lime juice
- Salt and black pepper
- 1 cup couscous, cooked
- 1 teaspoon lime zest
- ¼ cup toasted pumpkin seeds

- 1 cup fresh spinach, chopped
- 1 (15.5 ounce) can kidney beans, rinsed and drained
- 1 (14 to 16 ounce) block tofu, diced
- 2 summer squashes, diced
- 3 spring onions, quartered

**Directions**:

1. In a saucepan, heat 2 tablespoons oil and add oregano over medium heat.
2. After 30 seconds add parsley, chili pepper, cilantro, lime juice, 2 tablespoons water, vinegar, salt and black pepper.
3. Mix well then blend in a blender.
4. Add the remining oil, pumpkin seeds, beans and spinach and cook for 3 minutes.
5. Stir in couscous and adjust seasoning with salt and black pepper.
6. Prepare and set up a grill on medium heat.
7. Thread the tofu, squash, and onions on the skewer in an alternating pattern.
8. Grill these skewers for 4 minutes per side while basting with the green sauce.
9. Serve the skewers on top of the couscous with green sauce.

10. Enjoy.

**Nutrition**: Calories: 813Total Fat: 83gCarbs: 25gNet Carbs: 11gFiber: 1gProtein: 7g

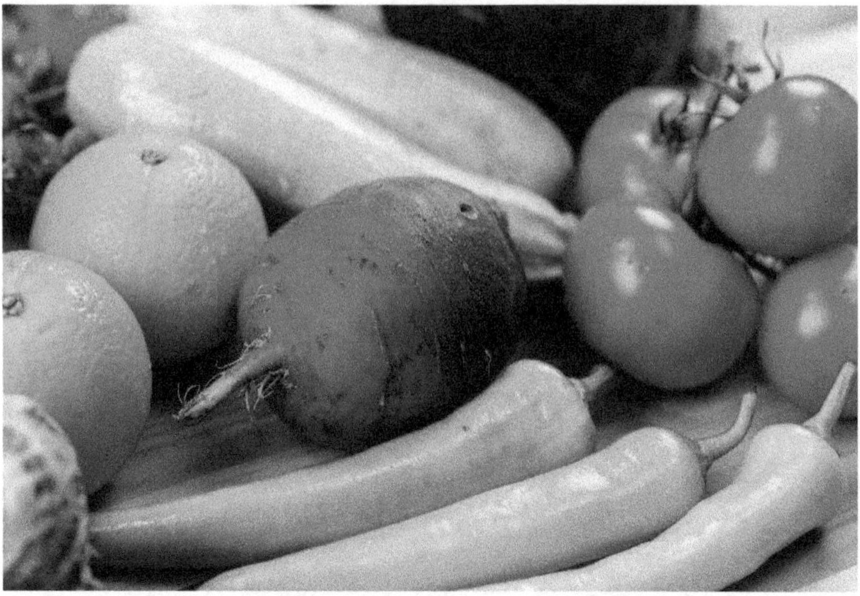

# SALAD

## 31. Lebanese Potato Salad

Preparation Time: 5 minutes

Cooking Time: 10 minutes

Servings: 4

**Ingredients:**

- 1-pound Russet potatoes
- 1 ½ tablespoons extra virgin olive oil
- 2 scallions, thinly sliced
- Freshly ground pepper to taste
- 2 tablespoons lemon juice
- ¼ teaspoon salt or to taste
- 2 tablespoons fresh mint leaves, chopped

**Directions:**

1. Place a saucepan half filled with water over medium heat. Add salt and potatoes and cook for 10 minutes until tender. Drain the potatoes and place in a bowl of cold water. When cool enough to handle, peel and cube the potatoes. Place in a bowl.

To make dressing:

2. Add oil, lemon juice, salt and pepper in a bowl and whisk well. Drizzle dressing over the potatoes. Toss well.
3. Add scallions and mint and toss well.
4. Divide into 4 plates and serve.

**Nutrition:** Calories 129Total Fat 5.5gSaturated Fat 0.9gCholesterol 0mgSodium 158mgTotal Carbohydrate 18.8gDietary Fiber 3.2g

Total Sugars 1.6gProtein 2.2gVitamin D 0mcgCalcium 22mg

Iron 1mgPotassium 505mg

## 32. Chickpea and Spinach Salad

Preparation Time: 5 minutes

Cooking Time: 0 minutes

Servings: 4

**Ingredients:**

- 2 cans (14.5 ounces each) chickpeas, drained, rinsed
- 7 ounces' vegan feta cheese, crumbled or chopped
- 1 tablespoon lemon juice
- 1/3 -½ cup olive oil
- ½ teaspoon salt or to taste
- 4-6 cups spinach, torn
- ½ cup raisins
- 2 tablespoons honey
- 1-2 teaspoons ground cumin
- 1 teaspoon chili flakes

**Directions:**

1. Add cheese, chickpeas and spinach into a large bowl.
2. To make dressing: Add rest of the ingredients into another bowl and mix well.
3. Pour dressing over the salad. Toss well and serve.

**Nutrition:** Calories 822Total Fat 42.5gSaturated Fat 11.7gCholesterol 44mgSodium 910mgTotal Carbohydrate 89.6gDietary Fiber 19.7g Total Sugars 32.7gProtein 29gVitamin D 0mcgCalcium 417mgIron 9mgPotassium 1347mg

# GRAINS

## 33. Indian Tomato and Garbanzo Stew

Preparation Time: 15 minutes

Cooking Time: 50 minutes

Servings: 4 to 6

**Ingredients**:

- 1 large onion, quartered and thinly sliced
- 1-inch fresh ginger, peeled and minced
- 2 cloves garlic, peeled and minced
- 1 teaspoon curry powder
- 1 teaspoon cumin seeds
- 1 teaspoon black mustard seeds
- 1 teaspoon coriander seeds,
- 1½ pounds (680 g) tomatoes, deseeded and puréed
- 1 red bell pepper, cut into ½-inch dice
- 1 green bell pepper, cut into ½-inch dice
- 3 cups cooked garbanzo beans
- 1 tablespoon garam masala
- 1/3 cup water

**Directions:**

1. Heat the water in a medium saucepan over medium-low heat. Add the onion, ginger, garlic, curry powder, and seeds to the pan. Sauté for about 10 minutes, or until the onion is tender, stirring frequently.
2. Add the tomatoes and simmer, uncovered, for 10 minutes. Add the peppers and garbanzo beans. Reduce the heat. Cover and simmer for 30 minutes, stirring occasionally. Stir in the garam masala and serve.

**Nutrition:** calories: 100fat: 1.2gcarbs: 20.9gprotein: 5.1gfiber: 7.0g

## 34. Simple Baked Navy Beans

Preparation Time: 10 minutes

Cooking Time: 2½ to 3 hours

Servings: 8

**Ingredients:**

- 1½ cups navy beans
- 8 cups water
- 1 bay leaf
- ½ cup finely chopped green bell pepper
- ½ cup finely chopped onion
- 1 teaspoon minced garlic
- ½ cup unsweetened tomato purée
- 3 tablespoons molasses
- 1 tablespoon fresh lemon juice

**Directions**:

1. Preheat the oven to 300°F (150°C).
2. Place the beans and water in a large pot, along with the bay leaf, green pepper, onion and garlic. Cover and cook for 1½ to 2 hours, or until the beans are softened. Remove from the heat and drain, reserving the cooking liquid. Discard the bay leaf.
3. Transfer the mixture to a casserole dish with a cover. Stir in the remaining ingredients and 1 cup of the reserved cooking liquid. Bake in the oven for 1 hour,

covered. Stir occasionally during baking and add a little more cooking liquid if needed to keep the beans moist.

4. Serve warm.

**Nutrition:** calories: 162 fat: 0.6gcarbs: 31.3gprotein: 9.1gfiber: 6.4g

# LEGUMES

## 35. Black Bean Buda Bowl

Preparation Time: 10 minutes

Cooking Time: 10 minutes

Servings: 4

**Ingredients:**

- 1/2-pound black beans, soaked overnight and drained
- 2 cups brown rice, cooked
- 1 medium-sized onion, thinly sliced
- 1 cup bell pepper, seeded and sliced
- 1 jalapeno pepper, seeded and sliced
- 2 cloves garlic, minced
- 1 cup arugula
- 1 cup baby spinach
- 1 teaspoon lime zest
- 1 tablespoon Dijon mustard
- 1/4 cup red wine vinegar
- 1/4 cup extra-virgin olive oil
- 2 tablespoons agave syrup
- Flaky sea salt and ground black pepper, to taste
- 1/4 cup fresh Italian parsley, roughly chopped

**Directions**

1. Cover the soaked beans with a fresh change of cold water and bring to a boil. Let it boil for about 10 minutes. Turn the heat to a simmer and continue to cook for 50 to 55 minutes or until tender.
2. To serve, divide the beans and rice between serving bowls; top with the vegetables.
3. A small mixing dish thoroughly combines the lime zest, mustard, vinegar, olive oil, agave syrup, salt and pepper. Drizzle the vinaigrette over the salad.
4. Garnish with fresh Italian parsley. Bon appétit!

**Nutrition**: Calories: 365; Fat: 14.1g; Carbs: 45.6g; Protein: 15.5g

# BREAD & PIZZA

## 36. Cornbread Waffles

Preparation Time: 6 Minutes

Cooking Time: 10 Minutes

Servings: 5

**Ingredients:**

- 1/3cup unsweetened plant-based milk
- 1 teaspoon apple cider vinegar
- 1/2 teaspoon baking powder
- 1/2 teaspoon baking soda
- 1 cup fine cornmeal
- 1/2 cup masa
- 1 cup unbleached all-purpose flour
- 1/3 cup unsweetened applesauce
- 1/4 cup sunflower oil
- Coconut oil cooking spray

**Directions:**

1. In a small bowl, whisk together the milk and vinegar and set aside.
2. In another small bowl, whisk the baking powder, baking soda, cornmeal, masa, and flour together.
3. Add the applesauce and oil to the bowl containing the milk and stir to mix.

4. Pour the wet Ingredients into the dry Ingredients and whisk until well combined.
5. Turn a waffle iron on and coat with cooking spray.
6. When the iron is hot, pour in enough batter to fill the waffle iron and cook for 4 to 5 minutes, or until lightly golden brown.
7. Take the waffle out of the waffle iron and cut it in half. Repeat with the remaining batter

**Nutrition:** Calories 175, Carbs 2.5g, Fat 9.5g, Protein 5.7g

# SOUP AND STEW

## 37. Roasted Red Pepper and Butternut Squash Soup

Preparation Time: 10 minutes

Cooking Time: 45 minutes

Servings: 6

**Ingredients**:

- 1 small butternut squash
- 1 tablespoon olive oil
- 1 teaspoon sea salt
- 2 red bell peppers
- 1 yellow onion
- 1 head garlic
- 2 cups water, or vegetable broth
- Zest and juice of 1 lime
- 1 to 2 tablespoons tahini
- Pinch cayenne pepper
- ½ teaspoon ground coriander
- ½ teaspoon ground cumin
- Toasted squash seeds (optional)

**Directions:**

1. Preparing the ingredients.
2. Preheat the oven to 350°f.
3. Prepare the squash for roasting by cutting it in half lengthwise, scooping out the seeds, and poking holes in the flesh with a fork. Reserve the seeds if desired.
4. Rub a small amount of oil over the flesh and skin, rub with a bit of sea salt and put the halves skin-side down in a large baking dish. Put it in the oven while you prepare the rest of the vegetables.
5. Prepare the peppers the same way, except they do not need to be poked.
6. Slice the onion in half and rub oil on the exposed faces. Slice the top off the head of garlic and rub oil on the exposed flesh.
7. After the squash has cooked for 20 minutes, add the peppers, onion, and garlic, and roast for another 20 minutes. Optionally, you can toast the squash seeds by putting them in the oven in a separate baking dish 10 to 15 minutes before the vegetables are finished.
8. Keep a close eye on them. When the vegetables are cooked, take them out and let them cool before handling them. The squash will be very soft when poked with a fork.
9. Scoop the flesh out of the squash skin into a large pot (if you have an immersion blender) or into a blender.
10. Chop the pepper roughly, remove the onion skin and chop the onion roughly, and squeeze the garlic cloves out of the head, all into the pot or blender. Add the water, the lime zest

and juice, and the tahini. Purée the soup, adding more water if you like, to your desired consistency. Season with the salt, cayenne, coriander, and cumin. Serve garnished with toasted squash seeds (if using).

**Nutrition:** calories: 156protein: 4gtotal fat: 7gsaturated fat: 11g

carbohydrates: 22gfiber: 5g

## 38. Cauliflower Spinach Soup

Preparation Time: 30 minutes

Cooking Time: 25 minutes

Servings: 5

**Ingredients:**

- 1/2 cup unsweetened coconut milk
- 5 oz fresh spinach, chopped
- 5 watercress, chopped
- 8 cups vegetable stock
- 1 lb cauliflower, chopped
- Salt

**Directions:**

1. Add stock and cauliflower in a large saucepan and bring to boil over medium heat for 15 minutes.
2. Add spinach and watercress and cook for another 10 minutes.
3. Remove from heat and puree the soup using a blender until smooth.
4. Add coconut milk and stir well. Season with salt.
5. Stir well and serve hot.

**Nutrition:** Calories: 271 kcalFat: 3.7gCarbs: 54gProteins: 6.5g

# SAUCES, DRESSINGS & DIP

## 39. Cilantro Coconut Pesto

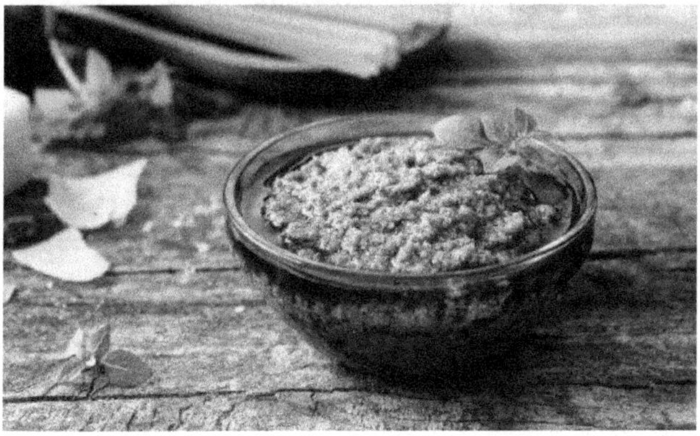

Preparation Time: 5 minutes

Cooking Time: 0 minutes

Servings: 2

**Ingredients:**

- 1 (13.5-ounce / 383-g) can unsweetened coconut milk
- 2 jalapeños, seeds and ribs removed
- 1 bunch cilantro, leaves only
- 1 tablespoon white miso
- 1-inch (2.5 cm) piece ginger, peeled and minced
- Water, as needed

**Directions:**

1. Pulse all the ingredients in a blender until creamy and smooth.
2. Thin with a little extra water as needed to reach your preferred consistency.
3. Store in an airtight container in the fridge for up to 2 days or in the freezer for up to 6 months.

**Nutrition**: calories: 141fat: 13.7gcarbs: 2.8gprotein: 1.6gfiber: 0.3g

# 40. Fresh Mango Salsa

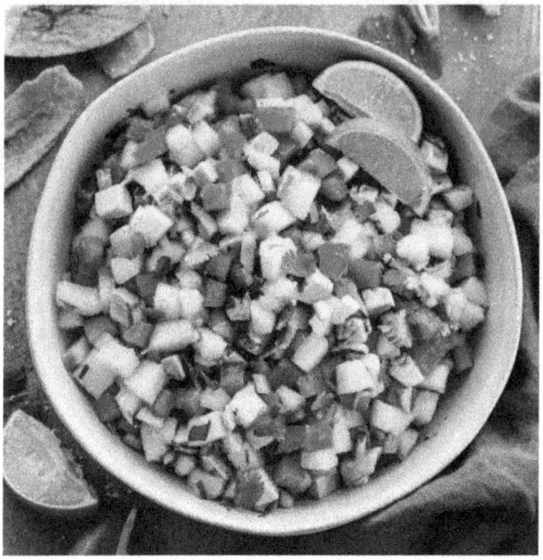

Preparation Time: 10 minutes

Cooking Time: 0 minutes

Servings: 6

**Ingredients**:

- 2 small mangoes, diced
- 1 red bell pepper, finely diced
- ½ red onion, finely diced
- Juice of ½ lime, or more to taste
- 2 tablespoon low-sodium vegetable broth
- Handful cilantro, chopped
- Freshly ground black pepper, to taste
- Salt, to taste (optional)

**Directions:**

1. Stir together all the ingredients in a large bowl until well incorporated.
2. Taste and add more lime juice or salt, if needed.
3. Store in an airtight container in the fridge for up to 5 days.

**Nutrition:** calories: 86fat: 1.9g carbs: 13.3gprotein: 1.2gfiber: 0.9g

# APPETIZER

## 41. Sesame- Wonton Crisps

Preparation time: 15 minutes

Cooking time: 10 minutes

Servings: 12

**Ingredients:**

- 12 Vegan Wonton Wrappers
- 2 tablespoons toasted sesame oil
- 12 shiitake mushrooms, lightly rinsed, patted dry, stemmed, and cut into 1/4-inch slices
- 4 snow peas, trimmed and cut crosswise into thin slivers
- 1 teaspoon soy sauce
- 1 tablespoon fresh lime juice
- ½ teaspoon brown sugar
- 1 medium carrot, shredded
- Toasted sesame seeds or black sesame seeds, if available

**Directions:**

1. Preheat the oven to 350°F. Oil a baking sheet and set aside. Brush the wonton wrappers with 1 tablespoon of the sesame oil and arrange on the baking sheet.
2. Bake until golden brown and crisp within 5 minutes. Set aside to cool. (Alternately, you can tuck the wonton

wrappers into mini-muffin tins to create cups for the filling. Brush with sesame oil and bake them until crisp.)

3. In a large skillet, heat the extra olive oil over medium heat. Add the mushrooms and cook until softened. Stir in the snow peas and the soy sauce and cook for 30 seconds. Set aside to cool.
4. In a large bowl, combine the lime juice, sugar, and remaining 1 tablespoon sesame oil. Stir in the carrot and cooled shiitake mixture.
5. Top each wonton crisp with a spoonful of the shiitake mixture. Sprinkle with sesame seeds and arrange on a platter to serve.

**Nutrition:** Calories: 88 Carbs: 14g Fat: 2g Protein: 3g

## 42. Macadamia-Cashew Patties

Preparation time: 15 minutes

Cooking time: 10 minutes

Servings: 4

**Ingredients:**

- ¾ cup chopped macadamia nuts
- ¾ cup chopped cashews
- 1 medium carrot, grated
- 1 small onion, chopped
- 1 garlic clove, minced
- 1 jalapeño or another green chili, seeded and minced
- ¾ cup old-fashioned oats
- ¾ cup dry unseasoned bread crumbs
- 2 tablespoons minced fresh cilantro
- ½ teaspoon ground coriander
- Salt and freshly ground black pepper
- 2 teaspoons fresh lime juice
- Canola or grapeseed oil, for frying
- 4 sandwich rolls
- Lettuce leaves and condiment of choice

Directions:

In a food processor, combine the macadamia nuts, cashews, carrot, onion, garlic, chili, oats, bread crumbs, cilantro, coriander, and salt and pepper.

Process until well mixed. Add the lime juice and process until well blended. Taste, adjusting the seasonings if necessary. Shape the mixture into 4 equal patties.

Heat-up a thin layer of oil in a large skillet over medium heat. Add the patties and cook until golden brown on both sides, turning once, for about 10 minutes in total. Serve on sandwich rolls with lettuce and condiments of choice.

**Nutrition:** Calories: 190 Carbs: 7g Fat: 17g Protein: 4g

## 43. Lemon Coconut Cilantro Rolls

Preparation time: 60 minutes

Cooking time: 0 minutes

Servings: 16

**Ingredients**:

- ½ cup fresh cilantro, chopped
- 1 cup sprouts (clover, alfalfa)
- 1 garlic clove, pressed
- 2 tablespoons ground Brazil nuts or almonds
- 2 tablespoons flaked coconut
- 1 tablespoon coconut oil
- Pinch cayenne pepper
- Pinch sea salt
- Pinch freshly ground black pepper
- Zest and juice of 1 lemon
- 2 tablespoons ground flaxseed
- 1 to 2 tablespoons water
- 2 whole-wheat wraps, or corn wraps

**Directions:**

1. Put everything but the wraps in a food processor and pulse to combine. Or combine the fixings in a large bowl. Add the water, if needed, to help the mix come together.
2. Spread the mixture out over each wrap, roll it up, and place it in the fridge for 30 minutes to set.

3. Remove the rolls from the fridge and slice each into 8 pieces to serve as appetizers or sides with a soup or stew.
4. Get the best flavor by buying whole raw Brazil nuts or almonds, toasting them lightly in a dry skillet or toaster oven, then grinding them in a coffee grinder.

**Nutrition:** Calories: 66Fat: 4gCarbs: 6gProtein: 2g

# SMOOTHIES AND JUICES

## 44. Chard, Lettuce and Ginger Smoothie

Preparation time: 5 minutes

Cooking time: 0 minute

Servings: 2

**Ingredients:**

- 10 Chard leaves, chopped
- 1-inch piece of ginger, chopped
- 10 lettuce leaves, chopped
- ½ teaspoon black salt
- 2 pears, chopped
- 2 teaspoons coconut sugar
- ¼ teaspoon ground black pepper
- ¼ teaspoon salt
- 2 tablespoons lemon juice
- 2 cups of water

**Directions:**

1. Place all the ingredients in the order in a food processor or blender and then pulse for 2 to 3 minutes at high speed until smooth.

2. Pour the smoothie into two glasses and then serve.

**Nutrition:** Calories: 514 Cal Fat: 0 g Carbs: 15 g Protein: 4 g Fiber: 4 g

## 45. Red Beet, Pear and Apple Smoothie

Preparation time: 5 minutes

Cooking time: 0 minute

Servings: 2

**Ingredients:**

- 1/2 of medium beet, peeled, chopped
- 1 tablespoon chopped cilantro
- 1 orange, juiced
- 1 medium pear, chopped
- 1 medium apple, cored, chopped
- 1/4 teaspoon ground black pepper
- 1/8 teaspoon rock salt
- 1 teaspoon coconut sugar
- 1/4 teaspoons salt
- 1 cup of water

**Directions:**

1. Place all the ingredients in the order in a food processor or blender and then pulse for 2 to 3 minutes at high speed until smooth.
2. Pour the smoothie into two glasses and then serve.

**Nutrition:** Calories: 132 Cal Fat: 0 g Carbs: 34 g Protein: 1 g Fiber: 5 g

# DESSERTS

## 46. Raisin Oat Cookies

Preparation time: 15 minutes

Cooking time: 8-10 minutes

Servings: 24 cookies

**Ingredients:**

- 1/3 cup almond butter
- ½ cup maple sugar
- ¼ cup unsweetened applesauce
- 1 teaspoon vanilla extract
- 1/3 cup sorghum flour
- 2/3 cups oat flour
- ½ teaspoon baking soda
- ½ cup raisins
- 1 cup rolled oats
- ½ teaspoon ground cinnamon
- ¼ teaspoon salt, optional

**Directions**:

1. Warm your oven to 350°F. Line two baking sheets with parchment paper. Whisk together the almond butter, maple sugar, and applesauce in a large bowl until smooth.
2. Mix in the remaining ingredients and keep whisking until a stiff dough form.

3. Divide and roll the dough into 24 small balls, then arrange the balls in the baking sheets. Keep a little space between each two balls. Bash them with your hands to make them form like cookies.
4. Bake in the preheated oven for 9 minutes or until crispy. Flip the cookies halfway through the cooking time. Remove them from the oven and allow to cool for 10 minutes before serving.

**Nutrition:** Calories: 115 Carbs: 14g Fat: 6g Protein: 2g

## 47. Oat Scones

Preparation time: 15 minutes

Cooking time: 22 minutes

Servings: 12 scones

**Ingredients:**

- 1 teaspoon apple cider vinegar
- ½ cup unsweetened soy milk
- 1 teaspoon vanilla extract
- 3 cups oat flour
- 2 tablespoons baking powder
- ½ cup maple sugar
- ½ teaspoon salt, optional
- 1/3 cup almond butter
- ½ cup unsweetened applesauce

**Directions:**

1. Warm your oven to 350°F. Line a baking sheet with parchment paper. Combine cider vinegar and soy milk in a bowl. Stir to mix well. Let stand for a few minutes to curdle, then mix in the vanilla.
2. Combine the flour, baking powder, sugar, and salt (if desired) in a second bowl. Stir to mix well. Combine the almond butter and applesauce in a third bowl. Stir to mix well.
3. Gently fold the applesauce mixture in the flour mixture, then stir in the milk mixture.

4. Scoop the mixture on the baking sheet with an ice-cream scoop to make 12 scones. Drizzle them with a touch of water.
5. Bake in the preheated oven within 22 minutes or until puffed and lightly browned. Flip the scones halfway through the cooking time.
6. Remove them from the oven and allow to cool for 10 minutes before serving.

**Nutrition:** Calories: 177 Fat: 6.0g Carbs: 26.6g Protein: 5.4g

## 48. Crispy Graham Crackers

Preparation time: 30 minutes

Cooking time: 11 minutes

Servings: 12

**Ingredients:**

- 1½ cups spelt flour, plus additional for dusting
- ½ teaspoon baking soda
- ¼ cup date sugar
- 1 teaspoon ground cinnamon
- ½ teaspoon salt, optional
- 2 tablespoons molasses
- 1 teaspoon vanilla extract
- ¼ cup unsweetened applesauce
- 1 tablespoon ground flaxseeds
- ¼ cup unsweetened soy milk
- 1 tablespoon maple sugar

**Directions:**

1. Warm your oven to 350°F. Line a baking sheet with parchment paper.
2. Combine the flour, baking soda, date sugar, ½ teaspoon of the cinnamon, and salt (if desired) in a large bowl. Stir to combine well.
3. Create a well in the middle of your flour mixture, then add the molasses, vanilla, and applesauce to the well. Whisk to combine.

4. Mix in the flaxseeds and soy milk, then knead the mixture to form a smooth dough. Add a dash of water if necessary.
5. On a clean work surface, dust with a touch of flour, then flatten the dough into a 1/8-inch-thick rectangle with a rolling pin on this surface.
6. Cut the dough into 8 equal-sized rectangles to make the crackers, then arrange the crackers on the baking sheet.
7. Sprinkle the crackers with maple sugar and remaining cinnamon. Poke holes into each cracker with a fork.
8. Bake in the preheated oven for 11 minutes or until crispy and golden brown. Flip the crackers halfway through your cooking time.
9. Remove them from the oven and allow to cool for 10 minutes before serving.

**Nutrition:** Calories: 120 Carbs: 20g Fat: 3g Protein: 2g

# 49. Overnight Oats

Preparation time: 5 minutes

Cooking time: 5 minutes

Servings: 1

**Ingredients:**

- ½ cup rolled oats
- 1 tablespoon ground flaxseeds
- 1 tablespoon maple syrup
- ¼ teaspoon ground cinnamon
- Topping Options:
- 1 pear, chopped, and 1 tablespoon cashews
- 1 apple, chopped, and 1 tablespoon walnuts
- 1 banana, sliced, and 1 tablespoon peanut butter
- 1 cup sliced grapes and 1 tablespoon sunflower seeds
- 1 cup berries and 1 tablespoon unsweetened coconut flakes
- 2 tablespoons raisins and 1 tablespoon hazelnuts
- 2 tablespoons dried cranberries and 1 tablespoon pumpkin seeds

Directions:

1. Combine the ground flaxseeds, oats, cinnamon, and maple syrup in a bowl, then pour the water into the bowl to submerge. Stir to mix well.
2. Leave them to soak within at least 1 hour, or overnight, then serve with the topping you choose.

**Nutrition:** Calories: 244 Fat: 16.0g Carbs: 10.0g Protein: 7.0g

## 50. Golden Muffins

Preparation time: 15 minutes

Cooking time: 30 minutes

Servings: 6

**Ingredients:**

- 1 orange, peeled
- 2 tablespoons chopped dried apricots
- 1 carrot, coarsely chopped
- 2 tablespoons almond butter
- ¼ cup unsweetened almond milk
- 2 tablespoons ground flaxseeds
- 3 tablespoons molasses
- ½ teaspoon ground cinnamon
- ¼ teaspoon ground nutmeg
- ½ teaspoon ground ginger
- 1 teaspoon apple cider vinegar
- 1 teaspoon vanilla extract
- ¼ teaspoon allspice
- ¾ cup rolled oats
- ½ teaspoon baking soda
- 1 teaspoon baking powder
- 2 tablespoons raisins
- 2 tablespoons sunflower seeds

**Directions**:

1. Warm your oven to 350°F. Prepare a 6-cup muffin tin lined using parchment paper.
2. Add the orange, apricots, carrot, almond butter, almond milk, flaxseeds, molasses, cinnamon, nutmeg, ginger, vinegar, vanilla, and allspice to a food processor and process until creamy and smooth.
3. Add the rolled oats to a blender and pulse until well ground. Combine the ground oat with baking soda and baking powder in a bowl. Stir to mix well.
4. Pour the orange mixture in the oat mixture, then mix in the raisins and sunflower seeds. Stir to mix well.
5. Divide the mixture into the muffin cups, then bake in the preheated oven for 30 minutes or until puffed and lightly browned. Remove them from the oven and allow to cool for 10 minutes before serving.

**Nutrition:** Calories: 287 Fat: 23.0g Carbs: 17.0g Protein: 8.0g

CPSIA information can be obtained
at www.ICGtesting.com
Printed in the USA
BVHW091946060521
606650BV00011B/1478

9 781801 832793